I0420189

Enzymes: An Easy To Understand Guide On Digestive Enzymes And The Vital Functions They Perform In Your Body

Disclaimer and Terms of Use: Effort has been made to ensure that the information in this book is accurate and complete, however, the author and the publisher do not warrant the accuracy of the information, text and graphics contained within the book due to the rapidly changing nature of science, research, known and unknown facts and internet. The Author and the publisher do not hold any responsibility for errors, omissions or contrary interpretation of the subject matter herein. This book is presented solely for motivational and informational purposes only.

Table of Contents

Introduction 4

Introduction

There are many substances and compounds that allow the human body to function properly. One of the vital substances is the enzymes which sustain life through their metabolic process. Enzymes are large biological molecules that are protein in nature. Enzymes work as catalysts in the body accelerating the metabolic reactions like the digestion. Since the enzymes are protein in nature, they contain several amino acids that are joined together. The enzymes in the body work on a specific substance called substrate (the substrate is used to give the enzyme its name). The enzymes are vital in the body as they help in the reconstruction, synthesizing, delivering, dispensing and eliminating the chemicals and ingredients that our bodies use on a day to day basis.

Digestive Enzymes

The digestive enzymes are the major category of the enzymes. Digestive enzymes are enzymes that are used to breakdown the macromolecules in the body into small building blocks that can be absorbed easily in the body. In the human body, the enzymes are found in the digestive tract and in the cells where they maintain the survival of the cells and also facilitate the proper digestion.

Since the human digestion starts in the mouth and ends in the small intestines, there are enzymes secreted in these specific areas. In the mouth the digestive enzyme is secreted by the salivary gland. In the stomach it is produced by the stomach lining cells, in the pancreas it is secreted by the pancreas exocrine cells and lastly in the small intestines it is produced by the secretory glands of the small intestines.

Properties Of The Enzymes

The digestive enzymes have different properties that allow them to perform properly;

- Enzymes are specific; one enzyme is used to control one reaction in the body. This means that the enzymes usually bind with only one substrate. There are three different types of specificity that are related to the digestive enzymes.

    1. Absolute specificity; the enzyme acts on one substance only

    2. Relative specificity; this is a property that allows the enzyme to act on different substances

    3. Stereochemical specificity; this is a characteristic that allows the enzyme to distinguish between stereoisomers.

- They are protein in nature;

- They are sensitive; they are easily affected by the temperature, pH and other factors

- They are catalysts; catalysts are substances that speed up a reaction without lowering the activation energy

- The enzyme can be regulated

- Some of the reactions of the enzymes are reversible

Structure Of The Digestive Enzymes

As mentioned, the enzymes are proteins and their activity is determined by their structure which is a three dimensional structure. The long linear chains of the amino acids are responsible for the three dimensional structure. The reaction that is carried by the enzymes takes place in the active site. Since they contain protein, most of the enzymes can be denatured (this means that the three dimensional structure will be unfolded and inactivated). The denaturation process may be reversible or irreversible depending on the structure of the protein (each amino acid sequence produces a specific structure which has different unique properties)

The Mechanisms Of The Enzymes

It is important for you to understand how the enzyme works. The enzymes usually attract the substrates to the active site by forming the enzyme-substrate complex. The enzymes then catalyze the chemical reaction a process that allows the products to separate from the enzyme surface.

The enzyme acts on the substrate in several ways which include;

- Lowering of the activation enzyme by stabilizing the transition phase

- The enzymes can lower the transition phase

- By providing an alternative pathway

- The enzymes increases the temperature of the process which in turn speeds up the process

Some of the enzymes require non-protein molecules to help them in the process. The molecules are usually referred to as co-factors. The co-factors can be organic or inorganic. Co-enzymes are also molecules that are used in the metabolic processes by transporting the chemical groups from one chemical group to another. The co-enzymes usually transport the chemicals that are not usually synthesized in the body but must be acquired from the diet. These chemicals might include; folic acid, riboflavin and thiamine. The co-enzymes are usually changed chemically due to the enzyme action.

Factors Affecting The Enzyme Activity In The Body

There are factors that might affect the activity of the enzymes in the body. The factors include

- PH; most of the digestive enzymes in the body are active under an optimal pH. Different enzymes have different optimal pH. When the pH in the body is extremely high or low, the pH activity might be slowed down as the enzyme might be denatured

- Temperature; as the temperature raises the enzyme reaction is usually increased. If there is any alteration in the temperature, the enzyme activity will be slowed down. High temperatures denature the enzyme as they interfere with the structure of the enzyme. When the temperature falls below the optimal temperature, the enzyme becomes inactive.

- Enzyme inhibitors; the enzyme inhibitors are substances that affect the enzyme action by altering the catalytic action of the enzyme. The enzyme inhibitors include; competitive, non-competitive and the substrate inhibitors. The competitive inhibitors represent substances that resemble the substrates are added to the enzyme active site. The non-competitive inhibitors are substances that are added to the enzyme active site to alter the enzyme so that the enzyme does not accept the substrate. The substrate inhibition on the other hand occurs when there are excessive amounts of the substrate

- The enzyme and substrate concentration also affect the enzyme activity in the body.

The Different Digestive Enzymes And Their Functions

The enzymes are broken down in terms of the place of secretion and the function. Since the digestion of the food in humans begins in the mouth, it is important to know the enzymes that are used during the digestion.

Mouth

The digestion begins with the breakdown of the carbohydrates in the food. The enzyme that is responsible for the breakdown of the carbohydrates is the enzyme amylase enzyme that is found in the saliva that is secreted from the salivary glands. The enzyme catalyzes the hydrolysis of the starch into sugars (disaccharides and the trisaccharides). Since the enzyme is specific, it can only hydrolyze the starch in to the above named sugars. The sugars are then converted into absorbable glucose by other enzymes.

Other uses

Apart from helping in digestion of the starch in the body, amylase has other uses that are of great importance.

- Enzyme amylase is also used in fermentation and bread making. After the enzyme has broken down the starch (which in this case is flour) in to simple sugars, yeast feeds on the simple sugars and then converts them into alcohol and carbon dioxide this causes the flour to rise. The enzyme is also used in the process of beer brewing.

- Can be used as a food additive

- Acts as an inhibitor of the alpha-amylase

- Amylase (bacillary) can be used in detergents

Stomach

In the stomach the enzymes that are used in the digestion are referred to as the gastric enzymes. The enzymes include;

1. Pepsin

The enzyme precursor is known as pepsinogen. The enzyme is usually released by the stomach cells. The enzymes are used in the breakdown of the proteins into peptides (short chains of the amino acids monomer). The pepsin enzyme is active under acidic conditions. This means that the enzyme can be denatured when the PH of the stomach rises to about 8.0 (alkaline). Some of the proteins that can be digested by the enzyme include; meat, eggs, milk and other dairy products. The enzyme however breaks down the protein partially into the small molecules, which are then broken down further by the pancreatic enzymes

2. Gastric Lipase

This is an enzyme that is secreted by the stomach cells. It is one of the acidic lipases in the body that don't require the bile acid to carry out its enzyme activity well. The enzyme is used to break down the short and medium chains of the fatty acids that are mostly found in milk. Once the fatty acids are broken down they are then moved to the small intestines

Pancreas

The pancreas is an organ that is responsible for the production of the endocrine hormones that are used in the circulatory systems. The pancreas also helps in the production of enzymes that help in the breakdown of carbohydrates, fats and proteins. The pancreatic juice contains all the enzymes. There are several enzymes that are produced in the pancreas

3. Pancreatic Amylase

The digestion of sugars (disaccharide and the trisaccharides) is done in the pancreas and the pancreatic amylase is responsible for the digestion. The sugars are converted to glucose which can be absorbed in the body.

4. Pancreatic Lipase (Pancreatic Triacylglycerol Lipase)

This is an enzyme that is secreted in the pancreas and is used to hydrolyze the fats in the body. The enzyme converts the triglyceride into monogylcerides and free fatty acids. The bile secreted in the body helps in the breakdown of the fat. The bile coats and emulsifies the fat droplets into small droplets which help the lipase to break down the fat easily.

5. Trypsin

This is a pancreatic enzyme whose precursor is the trypsinogen. The enzyme trypsin is produced in the pancreas in an inactive form. The enzyme is activated by the enteropeptidase which is found in the intestinal mucosa. Once the enzyme is activated it hydrolyzes or breaks down the peptide bonds. The proteases then further break down the peptide to amino acids making them to be absorbed easily.

6. Chymotrypsin

This is another digestive enzyme that is also a component of the pancreatic juice. The enzyme is active in the duodenum where it breaks down the protein to polypeptides through a process called proteolysis. The enzyme is secreted in its inactive form (Chymotrypsinogen) it is later activated to chymotrypsin.

7. Nuclease

The enzyme nuclease is a component of the pancreatic juice and it is used to separate the bonds between the nucleotides of the nucleic acid. The nucleic acids are the DNA and the RNA that are building blocks of the living organisms.

Small Intestines

The small intestine is divided into three parts namely; duodenum, jejunum an ileum. There are different enzymes that are secreted in these parts.

8. Sucrase

The name Sucrase is a name that is used to represent a number of enzymes that are used to catalyze the breakdown of sucrose to lactose and then to glucose. The enzyme is produced in the small intestines and also in the tips of the villi of the epithelium. Persons who suffer from sucrose intolerance usually experience the condition because the enzyme Sucrase is not secreted in the small intestines.

9. Lactase

This is one of the digestive enzymes that are mostly produced by infants and adult humans. The enzyme is used to digest the milk by breaking down the lactose to a simple sugar. Persons who don't produce the enzyme usually end up with the lactose intolerance condition. This means that the person cannot process whole milk.

10.   Maltase

This is an enzyme that is used to break down the maltose (which is a disaccharide) to simple sugars.

- The digestive enzymes help in the absorption of nutrients; the enzymes will catalyze the digestion process. This will enable all the nutrients to be digested and absorbed in the body.

- They help in the normal functioning of the body

- With the help of the enzymes the body absorbs the essential nutrients which help in providing energy for the body.

What Are The Factors That Can Affect The Digestive Enzymes?

There are times when the digestive enzymes don't work as they should in the body which might lead to serious problems in the body. There are factors that can cause the digestive enzymes to stop working as they should. Some of the factors include;

- Diseases; some diseases might prevent the digestive enzymes from working well. Cystic fibrosis, pancreatic cancer, acute or chronic pancreatitis, celiac and Crohn are some of the diseases.

- Low grade inflammation in the digestive tract

- Low stomach acid

- Chronic stress

- Aging

- Pancreatic insufficiency; this is the inability of the pancreas to produce enough enzymes for the normal functioning of the body. This condition can be caused by surgery, blockage of the pancreatic or bile duct

These factors might lead to the digestive enzyme deficiency in the body.

Symptom Associated With Digestive Enzyme Deficiency

If you have digestive deficiency you will experience;

- Weight loss

- Large amount of gas

- Feelings of indigestion

- Cramping after meals

- Floating, foul smelling, light colored stools

- You will experience frequent and loose stools
- Headaches

- Heartburn

- Slow recovery

- Stomach upsets

- Fatigue

- Low energy

- Allergies

How To Correct The Digestive Enzyme Deficiency

- Dietary interventions can increase the enzyme activity in the body. This is usually done by reducing the inflammation of the digestive tract. The diet can also help in removing the enzyme inhibitors in the body.

- Manage the conditions that cause the deficiency like the chronic stress.

- Eat food that balances the gut bacteria. The antibiotics and stress damage the gut bacteria.

Tips Of Balancing The Digestive Enzymes

- Adapt a Paleo lifestyle; the lifestyle incorporates eating the Paleo diets that have been reported to help in maintaining a healthy gut. The Paleo lifestyle, in addition to the diet, refers to having adequate sleep, having appropriate exercise and living a stress free life.

- Take the digestive enzyme supplements; the supplements will help you in regulating the enzyme in the body. As much as the enzyme supplements are beneficial to your body, they are not supposed to be taken by everybody. You will have to go to a doctor so that they can determine if you are qualified to take the supplements.

- Increase your intake of the fermented foods like the yogurts as they are good sources of probiotics. The probiotic bacteria help in proper digestion.

- Take the prebiotics; the prebiotics promotes the growth of the good bacteria in your body.

- Eating fiber will help you in reducing the constipation and digestion that usually cause the enzyme deficiency. The insoluble fiber that is found in the whole grains and the soluble fiber found in fruits and vegetables are beneficial in digestion.

- If you are on digestive enzyme supplement, it will be advisable for you to sprinkle the supplements in to your food if you cannot take the capsules.

- Chew your food well; this is important in promoting a functioning digestive system. Proper digestion will reduce indigestion. The carbohydrates starts to be digested in the mouth after the food comes in contact with the saliva

- Since the enzymes are found in the body and also in some fresh raw vegetables, fruits and nuts, it is important for you to eat the raw vegetables and the fruits. There are many creative ways that you can choose from when taking the fruits and vegetables; you can make the smoothies or eat them as salads. You should however eat the raw vegetables in moderation as some of them contain enzyme inhibitors.

- Legumes, grains nuts are some of the foods that can help in increasing the level of the enzymes as the contain enzymes and also because they help in fixing the gut bacteria.

- It is a known fact that the enzymes lose their activity level once they are in liquid form. If you are taking drinks, it is advisable for you to freeze the drink so that the enzyme activity level might not be affected.

- Preserve the enzymes in food by adding the nut butters and cooled chocolates. These are substances that are used to preserve the enzymes in the food for long.

- If you are pre mixing the food enzymes, it is important that you keep them cold so as to preserve the enzyme.

- Take the raw beets; they will help to reduce the toxins that build up in your body when your digestive process is not working properly.

- Including cinnamon in your meals will help you in supporting the bile flow

- Lemon and olive oil will also support a healthy bile flow in the bile and the pancreatic ducts.

- Drinking water 20 minutes before each meal will help you to hydrate your stomach hence promoting the production of the hydrochloric acid and increasing the flow of the pancreatic enzymes.

- Detoxification can also be very beneficial in the long run as it promotes proper digestion.

Ideas Of Foods And Drinks You Can Take To
Improve Your Enzyme Activity

Foods

- Honey
- Yogurt

- Maple syrup

- Peanut butter or cashew nuts

- Ketchup

- Pudding

- Brownies

Drinks

- Lemonade

- Milk and milk substitutes

- Juices

Digestive Enzyme Supplements

Many people who are affected by the digestive
enzymes deficiency end up taking the enzyme
supplements. The digestive supplements do improve

your enzyme activity however they are supposed to be taken in moderation. This is because it is very probable for some people to become dependent to the supplements. Some of the digestive enzyme supplements are the pancreatic enzyme supplements, lactose supplements for the persons with lactose intolerance and many more supplements. There are many reasons that can lead to the intake of the dietary supplements. The reasons include but not limited to;

- The enzymes are vital for the normal functioning of the body hence it is important to maintain the normal activity of the enzymes

- Some of the diets people take contribute to the reduction of enzyme supply

- There are factors in the human body that might cause the body to use the enzymes available faster

When it comes to choosing the right digestive enzymes supplements, there are a few factors you have to consider. They include;

- Quality and the price of the supplements; these are two factors that are closely relate. It is the assumption if a product is of low quality it will be cheap in terms of prices. So when it comes to choosing a digestive supplements that is good for you, you need to factor the price of the supplements.

- Consider the source that is used in the supplements; there are three sources that are used in the supplements. The three categories include; fruit sources, animal sources and the plant sources. The plant sourced supplements are the best and most stable supplements.

- Consider the ingredients used in the supplements. It is important for you to look at the label of the product before you buy it so that you see all the ingredients used.

- Consider the reputation of the company of the supplements. Not all the companies produce high quality products. It is important to research on the different companies before you choose the one to buy from.

- Consider the strength of the enzymes used in the supplements; different enzymes have different strengths and they perform differently.

- Consider the type of supplements you are to take; there are over the counter supplements and prescription supplements. The prescription supplements are supposed to be prescribed by a qualified physician. They are supposed to be used by the persons that have a medical condition like the pancreatic cancer

- Consider the dosage you are going to take; if you are not on prescription supplements, you will have to find a dosage that works for you. Some people take 1-2 capsules with their meals and others 4 capsules. The dosage depends on the quality of the supplements that you are taking.

Pros Of The Digestive Enzyme Supplements

- The supplements help in the regulating of the enzyme activity in the body

- They help in improving the immune systems. Once the enzyme activity in the body returns back to normal, the bile and the pancreatic enzymes start flowing in the normal rate. This will help to detoxify the lymphatic system (that is usually slowed down by the toxins that build during the enzyme deficiency)

- Help in providing you with energy as the nutrients will be digested and absorbed well

- The supplements help to improve your mood as some of the symptoms will be alleviated

Side Effects Associated With The Digestive Enzyme Supplements

Although the side effects associated with the supplements are not very common, some people who use the supplements have reported to experience some side effects.

- Stomach burning; this is usually caused by the over using of the supplements. Some of the supplements that contain enzyme proteases usually cause the stomach burning because of having excessive protease in the supplement

- Loose stools and excessive bowel movements; although this is usually associated with the enzyme deficiency, there are some supplements that usually cause the loose stools mainly because of the formula used in the supplements. It is rare for a supplement that contains a well balance formula to cause these symptoms.

- Bloating is another side effect that is associated with the dietary supplements; the bloating will occur after you finish eating your food. Although it is recommended that you take the supplements with food or after, it is advisable for you to take the supplements before eating food so that you can cope with bloating.

www.ingramcontent.com/pod-product-compliance
Lightning Source LLC
Chambersburg PA
CBHW061949280526
45787CB00004B/1782